Placenta:
THE GIFT OF LIFE

THE ROLE OF THE PLACENTA IN DIFFERENT
CULTURES, AND HOW TO PREPARE AND
USE IT AS MEDICINE

BY CORNELIA ENNING
EDITED BY CHERYL K. SMITH

Motherbaby Press

Eugene, Oregon

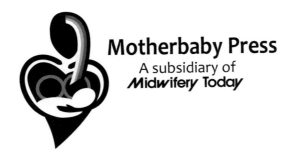

PO Box 2672
Eugene, Oregon 97402
www.midwiferytoday.com

Cover artwork: Eileen Somerday titled "for Love and Life."

Cover and interior design: Cathy Guy

Copyright © 2007 by Motherbaby Press

Notice of rights
All rights reserved. No part of this publication may be reproduced or transmitted in any form or by any means, electronic or mechanical, including photocopying, recording, or any information storage or retrieval system, without permission in writing from the publisher.

Library of Congress Cataloguing-in-Publication Data

ISBN: 978-1-890446-40-6

Printed and bound in the United States of America

Disclaimer: While the treatments in this book have been shown to be effective to the best of the author's knowledge, this information should not be substituted for medical treatment. Consult with a midwife, doctor or other healthcare professional before using the recommended treatments in this book.

The author and publisher do not guarantee the outcome of any treatments in this book and shall not be responsible for damages to people who choose to use the methods described in this book.

THE ROSE BUSH OF WALLONE

Once upon a time in Wallone, a district of Belgium, a young woman gave birth to a son. Her husband planted a rose bush in front of their house, as generations had done before. He buried the boy's afterbirth under the bush. The rose bush took root, nurtured by the afterbirth like the son once had been. Being carefully nursed by the parents, the little rose bush grew up to a magnificent tree and burst into full bloom. At the same time the son became a strong young man.

One day he left his family and stepped into the wide world. He instructed his mother to not worry about his traveling as a salesman in foreign countries. As long as his rose tree had green leaves and red blossoms, he would thrive as well.

His mother nursed and cared for the rose bush, enjoying the blooming roses every year. One morning, when she was about to 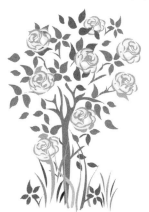 nurse her roses, her blood ran cold: All of the roses had dried out and the leaves had fallen off during the night. There was no life in the rose bush! Now she knew that her son had had a great misfortune.

The poor woman was carried, crying, into her house and put to bed to rest. For three days and nights she shed floods of tears, when finally a messenger arrived. He shared the bad news of her son's misfortune: Thieves had ambushed and murdered him in the dark of night.

Mourning her son, the old woman broke off the dried branch of the dead rose bush. As her son was buried, she put the branch below his feet.

In time new life came into the dried branch. United again with his "milkbrother" the rose bush grew new roots. The next spring tender buds sprouted above the ground and the following summer the bush brought a splendor of flaming red roses. Since then—year in and year out—a flood of red roses glows from the graves of Wallone.

CONTENTS

PREFACE 1

I. THE OLDEST TRADITIONAL REMEDY: PLACENTA   5

HISTORICAL AND ETHNOLOGICAL TRADITIONS 5
PLACENTA-TREES 6
THE CELTIC CALENDAR OF TREES AND PLACENTA 8
THOSE WHO KNOW ME LOVE ME 11
PLACENTA POTS 12
LUCKY CHARMS AND AMNION JEWELRY................. 14

II. BACK TO THE NATURAL HEALING POWERS OF THE PLACENTA   17

FAITH AND SUPERSTITION 17
THE MOST FEMININE OF ALL HEALING REMEDIES........ 18
MEDICAL USES OF PLACENTA........................ 23
USE OF PLACENTA IN COSMETICS..................... 26
A RETURN TO NATURAL REMEDIES 27
OLD TRADITIONAL KNOWLEDGE OF PLACENTA REMEDIES..... 29

III. MEDICAL APPLICATIONS   31

BREASTFEEDING.....................................31
NEWBORN COLIC 33
WHOOPING COUGH AND OTHER CHILDHOOD DISEASES 34

Diseases of the Heart and Circulatory System... 34
Menopause and Midlife Conditions................ 36
Hair Loss and Scalp Problems 39
Skin Conditions... 40

IV. From Placenta Birth to Healing Remedy   43

Methods of Preservation............................ 43
Fresh Placenta... 44
How to Process a homeopathic Mother Tincture... 46
Frozen Placenta... 46
Drying the Placenta.................................. 47
Further Processing of Placenta Powder.......... 48
application of placenta globules................... 50

V. Recipes for the Medicine Cabinet   51

Placenta Ghee (Mother Butter)..................... 51
Placenta Emulsion 51
Placenta Ointment 52
Placenta Tincture (Mother Essence)............... 52
Placenta Bath.. 53
Lactation Drink.. 53
Lactation Soup.. 54
Raw Placenta Pills 54

Placenta Capsules	55
German Postpartum Soup	56
Placenta Soup	56
Placenta Cream	57
Placenta Foot Ointment	57
Placenta Dressing	58
Compress	59
Nursing Oil (Placentolact)	59
Baby Care Paste	60
Hair Conditioner (Spiruzenta)	60
Facial Mask (Plastevia-Saluber)	61
Placenta Drink	61

VI. Women Tell Their Stories — 63

Does a Placenta Smell Appetizing?	63
Home Treatment for the Colicky Baby	64

VII. References — 67

VIII. Appendix — 71

PREFACE

As the number of facilities for cord blood banking has increased, professionals have argued about placenta remedies from a genetic viewpoint only. The pharmaceutical and homeopathic remedies from placenta tissues are similar to stem cells with their potential healing effects. They have had a long tradition in medical treatments around the world. Despite the fact that these products are available in some drugstores even today, most purchasers are not aware of their origin. The reason for this is that placenta products have been given more pleasant-sounding names, since modern people are supposed to think of the placenta as loathsome. Does this assumption about young parents' attitudes still apply today?

During their prenatal care consulting, midwives and doctors often answer questions about what to do with the placenta after the birth. The common practice in hospitals has been to dispose of the placenta like other unwanted body parts and medical waste. This practice is not followed by many young parents in certain parts of the world nowadays; in fact, just the opposite is true. The placenta is recognized as an infant organ with multifunctional duties: e.g., nutrition, oxygenation, cleansing of toxins and metabolism. Some parents claim the withheld body part, and in some countries the courts, and even legislative bodies, have given permission to do this.

Some parents and midwives see the disposal of the placenta by the healthcare facilities as a dispossession or even disrespect of their child. They question whether this body part can be adequately appreciated if it is treated as garbage. They believe, instead, that it should be treated with awe and respect.

Unfortunately, this view may put them at odds with the medical bureaucracy. In November 2005, a midwife in New York was suspended from her position in a hospital after she removed a placenta and buried it in her garden, upon request of the mother. The hospital claimed that it was "medical waste" and that she had violated their policy.(1)

On the other hand, Hawaii became the first state in the US to give women express permission to take their placentas home from the hospital after birth.(2) The outcry from native Hawaiians after placentas were legally declared infectious waste in 2005 came about not only because of their religious and cultural traditions, but because of fears that stem cells would be harvested from them without consent.

Looking at history we find the meaning of the old Middle High German word "placenta" is "mother's bread." In medieval times this word depicted the prenatal processing and nurturing as well as the cooking or baking of the placenta in the oven after birth.

Although remedies of placenta powder (PP), or mother essence, were well-known for centuries, they have become almost forgotten today. Until the end of the 19th century they were common in every European household and available in every drugstore. Our forebears still knew the remedies, which are manufactured from the "mother's bread" of a newborn family member. Not only was the baby a gift, but he brought a gift with him for all mothers, grandmothers and godmothers of the family.

Since 1990 old recipes for placenta ointments, homeopathy and Chinese medicine have been passed on in women's culture. Midwives, consultants and expectant mothers today look for information on the application of placenta remedies. More and more naturopathic therapists have come to recognize the power of placenta in complementary medicine like obstetrics, gynecology, pediatrics and geriatrics.

In the south part of Germany a few pharmaceutical manufacturers have produced placenta remedies since 1925. The market continues to grow, as long as the products are listed as containing not placenta but polypeptides. Many are aware of cosmetics, hair or skin care products with polypeptides.

Recently, drug manufacturers have met with more difficulties in obtaining the raw material as a result of increasing uncertainty regarding the placenta, such as:
- Who is the owner of the placenta—the newborn, the parents, the hospital or the researchers?
- Who is legally entitled to the placenta and products?
- What legislation exists regarding disease prevention and safe methods of sterilizing the raw material to produce placenta products?
- Do the customers really want to buy such products made of animal placentas or would they prefer other alternatives?

One alternative is to personalize placenta remedies. As raw material that is created and used by the same family, placenta is comparable to an auto transfusion prior to surgery. Undoubtedly, a placenta cannot harm the newborn himself. In addition, even his mother and grandmother may benefit from its healing power.

This booklet combines the experiences of midwives, doctors and naturopaths with our ancestors' traditions, and saves some old recipes from oblivion.

This booklet is written with the hope of reviving the traditional wisdom of the eldest remedy in "Herstory," with roots in development of the human race. Readers who have tried any of the recipes, can report their successes by e-mail to c.enning@t-online.de. Your contribution will add to the research of placenta remedies!

I. THE OLDEST TRADITIONAL REMEDY: PLACENTA

Historical and Ethnological Traditions

In medieval times the placenta was said to nurture an unborn child in body and soul. Its physiological functions during prenatal life paralleled its symbolic functions in postnatal life. Just as botanists today still call the two halves of a seedling that is changing into embryonic leaves the "placenta" of a plant, we find the same relationship between the human placenta in its amnion with the child. Even though they did not understand the function of a placenta as a biological filter, medieval people believed that the placenta allowed the fetus a certain degree of comfort—that it turned fetal imprisonment into a comfortable and bearable location. An unborn child was only supposed to lie there, so the placenta was also called "the bed of the child."

Indonesians describe an even more intimate relationship between the child and its placenta, calling it the "brother" or "sister" of the newborn. The Balinese expect that after death the placenta will go to meet them on their way into paradise.(3) In Java the placenta becomes a protector for mother and child.(4)

In Europe, until the end of the 18th century, the placenta was considered to be the other half of a newborn. Everything done to the placenta was supposed to affect the child before and after the birth. As a result, midwives left the placenta with the father, to avoid prosecution for child murder if they used the placenta for medical applications or buried it themselves.

In the years of burning witches after the protocol of the *Malleus Maleficarum* (a book published in 1486 to guide inquisitors in identification, prosecution and punishment of witches), most knowledge of midwifery was lost, including the art of placenta healing. Until at least the 19th century, however, midwives still understood, without the sciences of biochemistry or physiology, that the placenta is a remarkable part of the human newborn.

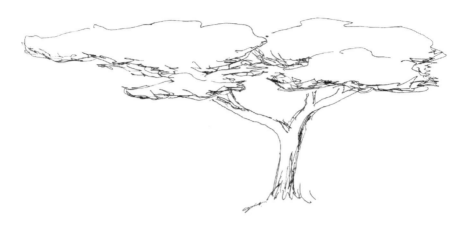

Placenta-Trees

According to Jacob Boehme's "doctrine of signatures" (the uses of a plant can be determined from some aspect of its form or where it grows), the tree-like shape of the placenta points to a similarity between the placenta and a tree. Even today many people and cultures worship trees as holy, destiny-weaving entities, bound tightly to the life of the human species.

"In all times the tree has been a well of inspiration and myths around the world. The roots make a tree a part of the chthonic world—the world of decay, out of which it draws its nourishment. The trunk is a mighty symbol of power and peace, while the annual change of leaves make it a metaphor for life: The flowering of youth, the wealth of maturation, the withering of old age and the decay when close to death. However, we always expect it to reburst into flower and to be forever renewing itself."(5)

Since the beginning of time people have had a special relationship to trees. The cosmic tree is the center of some religious traditions, because self-awareness is intimately tied to the understanding of trees. Cylinders from the Sumeric era (4000 AD) depicted people kneeling in front of a tree. In the centers of their shrines the ancient Germans built up a tree trunk or stilt as a symbol of the universal tree intended to focus the cosmic center. In every culture, the trace of tree life can be found in fine arts such as painting, songs and literature.(6) *Why did this universal symbol emerge in such a diversity of cultures, time and locations?*

The first perception of a human being is the prenatal environment of the womb with the silhouette of a tree. While floating in the amniotic fluid the fetus is shielded from the world by a spreading arch of branches. The placenta tree protects the fetus against impact and noise.

Films have been taken with microlenses of fetuses climbing up the cord to the disk of placenta tissue.(7) There they have groped at the hilly, smooth surface and some have even licked it like an ice cream cone. Frightened by noises, the fetus takes flight into the soft tissues between the vessel branches of the placenta. The head and ears are safe from the outside world (so sometimes babies turn into breech position when startled). In prenatal life the placenta is like a mighty, life-giving tree: the Tree of Life (Kabala).

Everyone is familiar with the shape of a tree. Respect for and worship of trees by people hint at our happy days in a prenatal paradise. Only this may explain why children who have never seen a real tree (e.g., they live in a treeless environment such as a desert) are able to draw trees. Children are also familiar with the image of a strong trunk, covered by a spreading roof, as their drawings show. The first emergence of the human being in children's drawings shows the character of a tree, too.

In many cultures the tree symbolizes the energy of life or even god. A "Holy Tree" is named and cared for, for example, the Ginkgo Tree in Asia or the Banyan Tree in Indonesia.

In some cultures a person's age is estimated by the growth rings of trunk slices from his or her birth tree.(8)

In Indonesia a special pot with the placenta is hung in the

branches of a long-living tree like the waringin tree, so that the newborn can benefit from the tree's blessed age.(9) The Placenta Tree, symbol for the life-energy giving placenta, accompanies us our whole life—from the cradle of the womb to our last resting place under the shade of a yew tree (preferred German cemetery tree) or cypress tree (preferred Turkish cemetery tree).

The Celtic Calendar of Trees and Placenta

Many parents are aware of the placenta's spiritual affinity with the life energy of the tree, according to an old European custom. They want the placenta to complete its life in dignity, after having provided nutrition and security for a long time. Parents of diverse backgrounds want to respect and appreciate the child's organ. As a symbol of gratitude many of them plant a young tree where they buried the placenta. The tree is supposed to soak up the placenta energy through its roots and transform it into fertile life-energy. As it grows to an imposing size, the tree attends to the newborn's development throughout childhood.

Every Ibo village in Nigeria is surrounded by a banana field. With the birth of a child a banana is planted and carries the name of the newborn. The village children own the field and use it as a special playground.(10) The trees are said to give fruits with future healing and nurturing effects on their protégés.

Ancient Germans expected the shadow of a birth-tree, as well as its size and shape, to make predictions about the path of life of his "milk brother."

The protective placenta tree of prenatal memories has become the postnatal consciousness of a "Tree of Life," which takes a piece of paradise into life on earth. Hermann Hesse considered trees to be symbols for memories, transition and rebirthing, as well as growth, instinct, natural life and fertility. "Nothing [is] more holy, more exemplary than a beautiful, powerful tree. Trees preach about the fundamental law of life."(11)

Stature and size of a tree depend on the plant species. According to Celtic tradition the choice of a tree for a newborn determines the map of life, like a horoscope. The holy tree creates a bridge between birth and death. Celtic myth refers to an apple tree as a symbol of completeness and of loving solidarity between humankind and nature, life and death, the netherworld and our world.(12)

The fruits of an apple tree were said to house the soul, awakening it to a new life. If a young woman ate an apple from a birth-tree, she was to become mother of a new human life. The souls of future beings waited for their bodily covering in the treetops. The word "apple" is derived from app-land, the Celtic Avalon. Since then, in many European countries an apple tree is planted after the birth of a child as the symbol of fertility and life energy.

A well-nourished apple tree, planted on a healthy placenta, is said to transfer this healing energy to the "milk brother" who eats its apples. To this day, gardeners learn about the transmission of qualities from one plant to neighboring plants.

For example, allowing a foxglove to grow under the shade of an apple tree is strictly forbidden, because of the absorption of digitalis through the roots. (The glycosides of digitalis are a common remedy against heart attacks.) The fairy tale of Snow White hints at this pre-Celtic knowledge: Eating the apple infused with digitalis causes the beautiful girl to fall into a deathlike sleep.

Almost all European people know about the tradition of burying the placenta under an orchard tree. Jacques Gélis, a distinguished French ethnologist, posited that this custom may have arisen from a desire to return to the realm of our ancestors, symbolized by the Family Tree.(13)

In some traditions, determining whether to plant an apple or pear tree over the placenta depends on the gender of the newborn. The apple tree is for a girl, the pear tree for a boy. In Switzerland the custom is to choose the apple tree for a girl and a nut tree for the boy.(14) The grandmother traditionally determines which kind of tree matches well with the individual newborn, because she has the richest fund of knowledge of life in the family.

Today with homebirths more common, the tradition of burying the placenta is still alive. Parents who live in a city without a garden look for an appropriate tree in the woods. They often choose a birch tree, intending to visit from time to time, to compare the growth of both child and tree. Until medieval times a placenta was buried under a birch, the tree of Freya, to worship the goddess of love with the sacrificial offering of "mother's bread." In addition, the newborn's cradle was carved of birch wood, representing chastity, light and renewal.(15)

Even today parents are supported by the Celtic tree calendar when considering the individual assignment of a tree species. According to this calendar the choice of tree depends on the date of birth, embedding it into the seasonal changes. The placenta tree calendar demonstrates in a pictorial, easy-to-understand way, the month and season in which a baby was born and simplifies choosing the proper tree of common wood.

By teaching the younger generation to care for an adopted tree that covers their life-giving placentas, parents have an opportunity to educate children about their responsibility for the woods on this earth.

The Celtic tree year starts with the mistletoe on December 24 and peaks at the equinoxes of spring and fall. The resistant oak, which still bears in winter's shortage, symbolizes the Summer Solstice. The mistletoe symbolizes Winter Solstice. The two halves of the tree disk are spaced regularly into seven tree beings.(16) The Christianized circle takes nine- to eighteen-day steps through the annual rhythm of nature.

Those Who Know Me Love Me

After the birth of the baby the placenta continues to function for a short while. The blood may take take up to two hours to stop flowing through the umbilical cord, which will then collapse. Our ancestors believed that a part of a child's soul stays with the placenta. Even after the placenta was born it performed its function as a root, as *thallus* (Greek for storage) and as fertile soil.(17) This is why it was never to be taken too far away from the child. The tree planted on top of it had to be in the immediate vicinity of the house.

In some areas the placenta was hung to dry inside the house or sacrificed to Odin's ravens by being hung from a tree. In Yemen the placenta is still laid out on rooftops for the birds to eat, which is believed to help the love between the new parents grow.(18)

In the cities, hiding the placenta underneath one's house used to be safer. The father usually buried it immediately after the birth, either in the basement or in an adjoining building, so the household could benefit as much as possible from the placenta's fertile powers.(19) In some areas a girl's placenta was buried to the left of the front door, a boy's to the right.(20) It was to be kept out of reach of animals and people or the fertility of the couple and other family members was endangered.(21) As long as the placenta stayed within the surroundings of the person it belonged to, no ill fate would befall him or her.

Being close to the placenta strengthened, in particular, the weaker children. The people of the Trobriand Islands (Pacific islands) bury the placenta in the garden to assure that the newborn will become a good gardener some day.(22) The people of the Batak tribes in Sumatra bury the placenta underneath the house or give it to the river in a tightly sealed pot of clay. This is believed to prevent the child from suffering from cold hands and feet later in life, which is considered a negative influence of the afterbirth.(23)

In Hawaii the placenta is "planted" following a secret religious ritual. The intent is to tie the child to the homeland so that he or she will not stray and will work on behalf of the land.(24)

As previously mentioned, in Sumatra and among most other Indonesian people the placenta is referred to as the younger brother or sister of the newborn.(25) A prayer of the Karo-Batak tribe in Sumatra says: Come here, my older and my younger brother (meaning the amniotic fluid and the placenta), who have been created together with me!(26) No one pays attention to the protective spirits in everyday life, but when danger exists they are called upon for help. They are believed to follow the person around and to be audible. They are man's brothers and affect "their" particular tribe members positively.(27)

In Nepal the placenta is called *Bucha-co-satthi* (the child's friend). The Mayans regard it as an older sibling. At times, when the growing child smiles unexpectedly the parents say he is playing with his older brother—the placenta.(28)

Placenta Pots

In 18th century Germany and France the newborn was to be handsome, smart and well-behaved in life if the placenta was buried close to the living quarters immediately after birth. Because throwing away the placenta was believed to lead to infertility in the mother, it was sometimes used as an attempt at birth control.(29)

In Sudan the placenta is viewed as the child's mental duplicate and is buried in a place that represents the parents' hopes and wishes for their baby. A Sudanese woman is said to have buried her son's placenta close to the medical faculty of the University of Khartoum, wanting him to become a doctor!

In many cultures of the world the custom of burying the placenta is still alive today. From the people of the Andes to the Indonesian cultures, burying the placenta under the home in a specially formed pot is still common practice. Just like the German women of the 17th and 18th centuries, these women are concerned about the child's soul suffering a painful loss by being separated from its nurturing, life-giving organ. Such pain was believed to impair the child's entire future development. Turkish women say this custom still exists among them, as well, and that it was introduced to them by the Arabs from the east.

The Institute for *Vor- und Frühgeschichte*"(pre- and early history) of the University of Tübingen, Germany, found pottery believed to have been hidden approximately 350 years ago. These vessels for the placenta had a special shape and had not been used for another purpose. They were decorated with patterns and sometimes with the owners' initials. Some of the vessels in Sindelfingen and in Boenningen had been buried upside down. This could be an indication of fear of spirits dwelling within the placenta. To keep these spirits from escaping, they had to undertake various protective magical rituals, including covering the vessels or turning them upside down.(30)

Several oral reports from the region of Heilbronn and the Black Forest indicated that knowledge has survived regarding customs surrounding the burial of the afterbirth, particularly in rural areas.(31) An exhibition in the fall of 1997 in Boenningen displayed various original placenta vessels and copies. Manos Nathan, an artist from New Zealand, where the custom of burying the afterbirth is still practiced today, has created a modern placenta pot, decorated with mythical figures. These are to remind us that humans come from Mother Earth, as well as from the human mother.(32) Soon-to-be parents can purchase these clay vessels for burial of the placenta.

Lucky Charms and Amnion Jewelry

If a child needs the special protection of a "double," even today in many areas of the world a dried part of the placenta will be tied around her neck. Most frequently a part of the umbilical cord or the amnion is dried and connected to a golden necklace or bracelet, sewn into the hem of a skirt or hidden in the school bag. Meaningful occasions, such as the first day of school or the examination for military service, are believed to have a better outcome if the young men carry a piece of their strengthening placenta twin with them. According to reports from the town hall of Backnang, Germany, one mother carefully stored the umbilical cord so it could be used as a lucky charm for her son later in life. She secretly sewed it into the hem of a piece of clothing to give him a number that would set him free when the drawing for the military service was done.(33)

In addition, the umbilical cord is believed to guarantee the child good manual and mental abilities. Those in the region of Franche-Comte, France, say of a mentally handicapped child: "It didn't carry its umbilicus in its pocket."(34)

The people of the Pacific Islands tie a knot into the cord before it has dried. Not until the child is able to untie this knot in the mummified placenta is he or she welcome to the community of adults. A similar meaning was attributed to the dried stump of the umbilical cord in Germany in the 18th century: Teachers judged the intelligence and brightness of a five- to seven-year-old child by how fast he was able to untie the knot.(35)

In Europe and Africa the dried cord was kept underneath the child's pillow or tied to the bed.(36) In Tanzania the cord is tied with a long black piece of cotton string, which remains wrapped around the baby's neck for 10 days. One Amazon tribe turns the cord into a bracelet decorated with beads to be chewed on when teething. The Australian natives make necklaces from the cord for the children, who wear them for protection from disease.(37)

The cord and the dried placenta seem to serve the same purpose. Some people of the world customarily dry a piece of the placenta until it is hard as a rock. Men then carry it in their pocket, wallet or belt at all times to bring about luck and money. In Tanzania the midwife's assistant buries the placenta in the courtyard, along with some salt and coins. This must be done in secrecy out of fear of the evil eye. Neighbors, envious of the expected wealth, could lay an evil eye on the placenta and endanger success.

If a baby is lucky enough to be born in the caul (with the membranes intact), the parents will keep a small piece of the amniotic membrane. They stretch the skin to be dried and paint symbols from religion, astronomy and nature onto the parchment-like tissue later. In Islamic countries parents most commonly choose "the eye of Fatima," whereas in Christian countries a picture of the child's patron saint is very popular. Delicate pieces of amnion are set in a pendant for arm and leg bracelets.

In Germany such paintings on the amniotic membrane

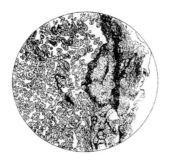 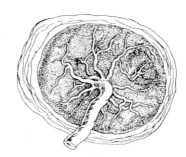

can be found in the form of window pictures or integrated in pieces of other art. Goldsmiths work it into necklaces and rings. No more personal a present can be given to a child for christening than a piece of jewelry with her very own amniotic membrane.

In some modern industrialized countries such as Germany, parents are familiar with the custom of retaining their child's placenta by having homeopathic pills made from a small piece of the placenta. Thus the placental powers the child had thrived on before the birth can still be used to strengthen him during childhood diseases or in dangerous situations. The placenta pills are a clean variation of the former soul mate and can easily be kept near the child. Many mothers still believe in the placenta's healing properties, just like mothers did 200 years ago. *Can these powers be explained scientifically?*

II. BACK TO THE HEALING POWERS OF THE PLACENTA

Faith and Superstition

Cultural habits subject to the taboos of sexuality and birth often are hard to explore. Written historical proof rarely exists; illustrations and other clues are more likely to be found. Sensationalistic reports on groups of cannibals supposedly eating a newborn's placenta as a birth rite have appeared in the press from time to time. Most of the time the men are said to have eaten the organ raw or cooked in order to improve their hunting abilities. De Levy reported on consumption of the placenta in 1556.

In 1884 Engelmann reported on the practice in Brazil and Russia. Around 1900 the placenta was said to have been eaten in Sudan. Schmaltz mentions pre-modern tribes practicing placentophagia to this day.(38)

These stories might be true, considering that the enzyme level of a placenta eaten raw could have strengthened the warriors' immune systems. Those who have experience with placenta therapy know that eating cooked placental tissue can cause euphoria.

The highly potent hormones that flood a pregnant woman's body can explain the rejuvenating effect of pregnancy, particularly on an older woman. One can see why during pregnancy many women experience a physical and psychological high they had not known before.(39) Scientists have discovered that the placenta contains hormones that inhibit stress and trigger the release of endorphins. The tribes mentioned by Schmaltz might have used the mood-enhancing effects for their hunting spirits.

Scientific research does not confirm travel reports of this sort, however. The likelihood of obtaining additional information on the customs and healing methods of so-called primitive people will decrease over time. The dwindling of their natural environments leads to their extinction and along with it the loss of their knowledge of placenta therapy. Thus we probably will never learn in what manner primitive people use their placentas today.

Like other mammals, humans have to detach the umbilical cord and protect the newborn from animals of prey. In a hostile environment that does not allow for longer periods of rest in one place, such as the prairie or the desert, the well-being of mother and child depends on a speedy recovery from birth. Consumption of the placenta can reduce the recovery period to a couple of days. Mothers in those regions of the world must be back in shape quickly to continue migrating with their tribe. In our present time and with our current lifestyles, a woman will also regain her strength very quickly if she eats the placenta soon after the birth. This is why some European midwives encourage new mothers to eat a little bit of the placenta, as well. To this day people still consume the placenta in some poorer regions of Europe, such as Poland and the Czech Republic.

The Most Feminine of All Healing Remedies

Less sensationalistic reports on the therapeutic use of the placenta come from China, South America and Eastern Europe. Into the 19th century, pharmacies were responsible for producing placenta remedies, as well as trading with them. Chinese women still sell their placentas to pharmacies today to earn some extra money.

A pharmacy at the market in Cousco, Peru, has a poster in the shop window asking its customers to make their placentas available after the birth. Until the end of the 19th century the pharmacies commonly sold placenta powder in Europe as well.(40)

In the 16th century a piece of the placenta was added to the mother's first postpartum meal in southern Germany.(41) The custom of offering a woman chicken broth with a piece of the placenta for her first meal after giving birth is still alive in many European regions.(42) A drink of white wine in which a piece of placenta had been preserved was believed to speed up the delivery of the afterbirth and control bleeding. If, following the prior birthing of a midwife's client, she had not prepared a concoction of wine and placenta, a drink was instead made of ground, baked placenta tissue dissolved in water. According to inventory lists "a jar of this powder" was kept in stock at all town pharmacies until the end of the 19th century. Not until the turn of the 20th century did use of the placenta powder gradually diminish.(43)

The religious ritual of sacrificing bread in church is an important clue to the use of placenta remedies in pre-Christian Europe. The mother used to take the placenta to church. At the altar of Mother Mary people prayed for better lactation of the nursing mother. To this day an altar for Mother Mary is still in every Catholic Church, despite passionate efforts to get rid of them. Countries that deem nursing the newborn unnecessary and where breastfeeding is seldom practiced consequently have reduced the shrine of Mother Mary to a statue in a side room of the church.

The shrines of Mother Mary in South America are particularly large, often even larger then the main altar itself, because they are the ones most frequented by the majority of the population. The bishops more or less tolerate, rather then support, the worship of Mother Mary as a pre-Christian custom.

What no longer exists is a placenta-blessing ceremony

or female priests healing with placentas. Around the world "civilized women" have lost their confidence in the shrine of Mother Mary. The link between the art of healing and religion is gone.(44)

The art of producing and applying placenta remedies was only lost partially during Christianization in South America and in Europe after the Renaissance. In only the poorest countries of the world has the worship of Mother Mary survived. Yet women still believe in the milk production-enhancing effect of their prayers to Mother Mary. Drying and pulverizing the placenta has been pushed to the privacy of their homes, where it is still known and often practiced.

According to a message from an Indian monk of the Dominican monastery of Lima, Peru, the statue is still believed to have the healing powers over a woman's fertility and lactation that were once attributed to placenta powder. This may be why many households own a statue of Mother Mary.

Little is left of the belief in Mother Mary's positive effect on fertility in some Eastern European countries. However, in areas distant from modern infrastructure, like Anatolia and Poland, traditional accounts tell of how a woman is to use the afterbirth. According to midwives from Poland, Turkey, Portugal and Spain, the placenta should be dried and pulverized and the powder applied both internally and externally. Even farther east—in Vietnam, Korea and Thailand—placenta hormones have always been used in folk medicine for the treatment of badly healing wounds, as well as for blood circulation disorders.(45)

Throughout the world generations have passed down knowledge of how ingesting placenta helps a mother's postpartum recovery. Women using placenta remedies after birth feel stronger, are happier and can breastfeed more easily. If edema, elevated blood pressure or traces of protein in the urine signal malfunction of the kidneys during pregnancy, placenta remedies can eliminate these symptoms quickly. The symptoms of toxemia in pregnancy usually go hand-in-hand with a late onset of lactation after birth. Swelling in the fingers and legs may take up to six weeks to disappear again. Placenta remedies, such as the powder, emulsion or an injection with the extract, can speed up this process considerably. With this treatment toxemic women can breastfeed well within two weeks. Traditional Chinese Medicine (TCM) uses placenta to strengthen the kidneys. Mood swings resulting from a drop in the blood progesterone level respond well to a treatment with placenta remedies. Many conditions during birth, the postpartum period and nursing would not arise if we returned to the old custom of applying placenta remedies.

The baby also may suffer consequences if a mother doesn't ingest her placenta. The newborn receives important hormones such as estrogen, progesterone and oxytocin with the mother's milk. Diamond assumes that the mother should consume the placenta not only for her own sake, but for the baby's sake as well.(46) Up until birth, the baby lives happily inside the uterus until the process of birth causes separation anxiety. If Mom eats part of the placenta, some of it may make it back to the baby and somehow contribute to a reunion. If the placenta is simply thrown in the trash, as commonly occurs, the baby will be deprived of this.

Diamond also noticed that many people were able to feel true love toward their mothers and themselves for the first time in their life after taking a placenta concentrate.(47) Humans need the hormone oxytocin to be able to feel love.

A baby experiences love for its mother as a result of the oxytocin in her milk.(48)

What Diamond expresses may have a biochemical foundation. Medical doctors and midwives have begun to scientifically study the correlation between perinatal bonding and the hormone levels of mother and baby.(49) A newborn responds to the elevated oxytocin level at birth with eyes opened wide. It looks at its mother the same way lovers have always looked at one another.

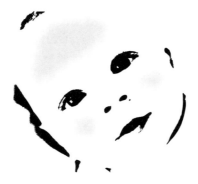

Human milk has a tempting sweetness—that is, if the hormone level is correct. A mature placenta contains a high level of oxytocin (often called the love hormone). Women whose milk lacks oxytocin because of toxemia, gallbladder disease or a stressful birth, can make up for it by using a placenta remedy.

Research on love is a significant factor in the scientific revolution currently taking place, which will greatly influence the 21st century. All scientific theoretical considerations point towards the major impact of humans' early experiences in life. This is particularly true for the time right around birth, which is crucial for the development of the ability to love.(50)

Medical Uses of Placenta

European Union

In the 20th century new laws were passed in Europe regarding the medical trade, some of which affected the use of placenta remedies in Europe. For example, laboratories in Germany are not allowed to sell any organic preparation directly to the consumer. The pharmacist, as a professional, must certify the remedy for purity, sterility and expiration date before it can be given to a patient according to the orders of a therapist. Doctors, midwives and health practitioners are allowed to work with placenta remedies as part of a therapy but are not allowed to give them out to patients. These laws are to guarantee that the medicine is safe for the patient.

Under German law, parents who plan to use their placenta for the preparation of remedies must find a therapist who will send their placenta to a suitable laboratory and who will prescribe the remedy competently. (See Appendix A for a sample form to order processing.)

Individuals who have the ability to produce placenta remedies and to apply them can process the placenta themselves. However, neither the raw material nor the finished remedy may be passed on to other people for therapeutic purposes.

China

Placenta has been used in Chinese medicine for more than 1400 years. It is believed to be an effective treatment for a variety of conditions, including infertility, immune system strengthening, asthma, liver problems, arthritis and many more conditions.(51) Some practitioners inject an extract of placenta to treat such conditions. They note that side effects can include increased temperature, itching and red spots on the skin. In addition, they recommend against teenagers using placenta remedies, because of the effects of estrogen.

Japan

In Japan placenta products are used for a variety of conditions. The placentas used are tested for hepatitis and sterilized. The resulting remedy is used for treatment of cerebral thrombosis and heart attack, as well as to build the immune system.(52)

Cuba

In the 1970s Cuba exported 40 tons of human placentas to a French laboratory after discovering that it could be used to successfully treat vitiligo, a condition that causes the skin to lose pigment.(53) The availability of this treatment in Cuba has brought patients from countries around the world.

Because of this demand, as well as an increase in medicines and cosmetics developed using placenta, a manufacturing plant was built during 1991-1995 to meet the need. The products are now used to treat not only vitiligo, but alopecia and psoriasis. Research indicated that placenta was useful in delaying the cell aging process.

United States

Placenta medicine is not recognized in the US, either in popular culture or law. As a result, anyone who would like to have placenta remedies created must do so themselves or risk running afoul of the Food and Drug Administration (FDA). Placenta can still be found in some cosmetics, but claims for its effectiveness are prohibited.

Russia

A Russian physician, Dr. Valentin I. Govallo developed a treatment for cancer using injected placental tissues.(54) His research showed that they suppressed lymphocytes from maternal tissues. He also noted that they caused transient fever, shivering and weakness. The treatment resulting from this research, immunoembryotherapy, has been used in Mexico, Bahamas and San Diego, California.(55) In Germany, doctors are also using placenta injections for treatment of cancer, AIDS and multiple sclerosis.

Mexico

In Mexico, women still use placenta as a remedy or preventive for various problems. Alison Bastien, a Mexican midwife, reports on a new mom who cut up bite-sized pieces of her recently birthed placenta and simply swallowed the chunks, one or two a day, to ensure good milk supply and strength. She swears by it and did it for a month postpartum. She froze the tiny chunks to keep them fresh and easier to swallow. At first she chewed them, but eventually found that swallowing them whole worked better.

Another use is placenta tincture in drops for six weeks to prevent post-operative depression as well as help with the hormonal changes after a hysterectomy. The tincture is also given to women with menopausal problems. Ten drops of the tincture directly on the tongue one to three times a day helps prevent hot flashes, mood swings, palpitations, etc.

Use of Placenta in Cosmetics

In the United States placental materials were first used as cosmetic ingredients in the 1940s. At that time the products were claimed to stimulate tissue growth and remove wrinkles. Under the law, these claims, as well as the fact that the cosmetics contained hormones, caused placenta-containing products to be classified as drugs. The FDA then declared them to be ineffective and misbranded.

This challenge caused placenta suppliers to change their marketing strategies. They claimed that the hormones in their placenta ingredients had been extracted and were no longer in the product. They then offered placental raw materials without medical claims—only as a source of protein. Currently, primarily cow and sheep (bovine and ovine) placentas are used in cosmetics in the US, although human placenta materials are not explicitly prohibited.(56) With the exception of colors and certain prohibited ingredients, a cosmetic manufacturer may use essentially any raw material in a product and market it without prior FDA approval. Marketing it as a drug, or remedy, is another matter.

In the 1990s researchers discovered that hair care products containing placenta were linked to premature sexual development in African American girls.(57) This was believed to be related to the estrogen contained in placenta. A study by Silent Spring Institute later showed that these products were much more likely to be advertised in magazines that were marketed to African Americans.(58) This finding of premature puberty in young girls mirrors the belief of the Chinese that placenta remedies should not be used by young people.

Some cosmetic manufacturers still use the estrogens of

the placenta in their products. The cocktail of substances in placenta remedies is believed to stimulate hair follicles. These substances have been used to treat hair loss and seborrhea. Amazing results have been achieved for "alopecia areata," circular hair loss, as noted in Cuban research.

In 1976 the use of human organs, including placenta, in the manufacture of cosmetics was banned in Europe. This ban was amended, but is still in effect, having been reiterated in a 1998 Opinion of the European Group on Ethics in Science and New Technologies to the European Commission.(59) The rationale was concern regarding Creutzfeldt-Jakob disease (CJD), a brain wasting disease similar to mad cow disease.

In Mexico some midwives use the placenta in some form (usually tincture) in facial beauty creams.(60)

Japanese cosmetic surgeons offer not only surgical treatments but placenta extract shots to treat wrinkles. The shots offered to men and women are different, with some of the female hormones removed in the men's.

A Return to Natural Remedies

All nations in the world have to minimize expenditures for medicine and therapy. That is why we are seeing a return to natural medicine by some in industrialized countries. People are becoming interested in old remedies of medieval times, as well as in medicinal herbs and natural healing methods.

Placenta remedies are organ-based remedies, which many still reject as unclean or nasty. However, in an era of excessive meat consumption, organ transplants and contaminated blood transfusions, this old taboo is decreasing. As we gain more knowledge about the causes of infectious diseases, remedies that we can obtain and process individually are becoming attractive again. Auto transfusion and bone marrow and skin transplants are becoming more common. More and more frequently doctors are using urine therapy and desensitization for allergies. Parents in particular are rediscovering the placenta, with all its healing powers.

The ability to inexpensively and simply obtain a placenta makes it even more appealing. Using placenta membranes to cover burns is by far less expensive than any other method used by public hospitals. The quick availability, the small effort involved in gaining access to it and applying it, the simple waste management when taking care of the wound, as well as the incredible results in the healing process of the burn are the great advantages of using the placenta membranes for a natural and biological dressing.(61)

Placenta remedies used by the person to whom the placenta belongs have additional benefits: They are not polluted by foreign bacteria and their composition is adjusted to the person's particular state of health and can be available for a lifetime. The use of commercial medicine may be unnecessary for many different treatments. Despite pollution and the threat of a water shortage, placenta medications are available as a pure remedy, as long as babies are being born. In addition, they combine well with other medication and treatments, sometimes increasing their effectiveness.

For the "family doctor" of the 19th century (62), when the housewife and mother had the primary role of healing and caring for family members, placenta remedies were a true treasure. This ancient knowledge should not be lost with the changing living conditions of today's families.

Old Traditional Knowledge of Placenta Remedies

The placenta nosode is effective for many diseases. The homeopathic globules of the cord have similar, but not equal, effects as placenta nosodes. Various diseases have been treated successfully in many countries for centuries.

Over the last 10 years many parents, midwives, pediatricians, homeopaths and health practitioners have accumulated interesting experiences with placenta remedies. Whether childhood diseases, gynecology, geriatrics, ophthalmology or general medicine—the possible applications are widespread. Only a few of these experiences have been documented and are accessible to the general population.

According to Traditional Chinese Medicine (TCM), placenta is considered a powerful and sacred medicine, full of life force. Raven Lang, a midwife who has studied TCM, advises women to use placenta during the postpartum period to aid in recovery from childbirth, prevent postpartum depression and minimize bleeding.(63)

III. MEDICAL APPLICATIONS

Breastfeeding

Taking the placenta as a powder, particularly in the first nine months after giving birth, is an old custom. It helps the uterus return to its original shape and size and speeds up the mother's recovery as well. It prevents depression, which can occur even after several months as a result of fluctuating hormones.

The powder is particularly useful for enhancing the milk supply. Within 20 minutes of taking a pinch of placenta powder, a breastfeeding mother will feel her milk coming in. Even women who haven't given birth themselves but want to breastfeed an adopted baby can get their milk to come in by taking the placenta remedy and putting the baby to the breast regularly. The dosage may have to be adjusted, as each placenta has its own potency. Some midwives who are experienced in counseling breastfeeding mothers can judge the individual dosage. Using too much of the placenta powder may result in engorged breasts. This problem is easily solved by reducing the amount of powder used.

The production of breast milk follows a natural daily rhythm. Women make the most milk at night which is when most babies also catch up on any unfulfilled daytime needs. Between 6:00 am and noon, most babies sleep for a stretch of roughly five hours without nursing. In the afternoon the milk supply lessens and the child nurses about every two hours. In the evening many babies are quite restless and try to get the milk production going again by sucking constantly. The flow of milk is rather low around 6:00 pm, when the mother starts to feel tired.

This circadian rhythm of lactation may cause a mother to worry that she cannot satisfy her baby with the available milk. Placenta remedies, particularly powder or homeopathic pellets, can help. Beginning at 4:00 pm the woman should take a pinch of powder or two globules of a low potency D2 every two hours.

The evening feedings will be spaced in three-hour intervals again. By 8:00 pm the mother will probably do fine without any more medicine.

Placenta globules can be helpful when weaning the baby off the breast, as well. Some babies wean themselves suddenly. The mother is then stuck with all the milk and may develop breast engorgement or even mastitis. Higher homeopathic potencies can suppress lactation rather quickly. If the treatment is combined with other homeopathic remedies the breast will recover even faster.

First-time moms, in particular, have had amazing success with placenta remedies during breastfeeding. To enhance their milk supply, they can eat a thin slice of the raw placenta for five days in a row.

Sometimes the milk supply will drop again once the mother stops taking the remedy and she will need to repeat the treatment. Because the placenta doesn't stay fresh for long, it must be frozen or dried. The mother can then take the placenta remedy as needed until her milk supply is reliable. Once she reaches this point, the baby will be able to sleep up to six hours straight at night. In turn, the mother will recover more quickly from the strains of labor and birth.

Lactation consultants and midwives frequently see moms with sore nipples due to the baby's inability to nurse efficiently. The underlying cause may be a weak let-down-reflex. Mothers can take the placenta remedy to help them "let go of their milk."

When a fever or childbirth injury needs treatment a combination of raw placenta and enzymes can be useful. These remedies work together well, augmenting each other and speeding the healing process.

Treatment with a combination of placenta and enzymes after a birth involving premature rupture of the membranes or stained amniotic fluid may prevent an infection. The placenta, as well as the enzymes, helps to produce more milk with no side effects for mother or baby. (Note: Fermented foods, such as yogurt or kefir, sauerkraut, pickles and kim chee, and "green juices" are good sources of enzymes.)

Newborn Colic

During the third week of life many newborns begin to have regular crying spells in the evening and at night. Often parents interpret this as a tummy ache. This is probably not all wrong, since new synapses are developing in the gastrointestinal system, transmitting information between nerves and the brain.

Professor Emeran Meyer, Chairman of the new Mind-Body Collaborative Research Center at the University of California at Los Angeles has done research on how messages from the gut get to the brain. To him, the digestive system is "the second brain." It has everything an integrative nervous system needs; one could say it is thinking.(64)

The newborn is very aware of these sensations because they are new. Not until the baby has become used to them—like one can get used to a scratchy sweater—can she start ignoring the signals. The baby's ability to tolerate stress may be affected by the mother's hormones at birth. Fear, stress and danger may lead to cramping of the intestinal muscles and to diarrhea. The tummy of a colicky baby may be in a state of alarm because of the stress experienced by the mother before, during or after the birth.

Likewise, the stress one is exposed to early in life is branded into the brain and gut and rules the sensitivity of the axis between the bowels and the brain for the entire life.

The negative affects of the mother's stress hormones during the delivery can be reversed in many ways. Various water therapies such as Watsu (Water-Shiatsu), Aqua Wellness, Baby Yoga and baby massage are helpful.

One way to enhance the benefits of early baby swimming classes is to give the baby love hormones (oxytocin) in the form of a placenta remedy. The baby will then remember the mother's love from the time before birth, just as he does when nursing at the breast. The homeopathic potency C7 of the placenta nosode has been shown by experience to be suitable for children. Alternatively, one can add placenta tincture (see page 65) or placenta powder to the baby massage oil.

Whooping Cough and Other Childhood Diseases

The treatment of childhood diseases can be accompanied by placenta nosodes. Placenta pills do not impair allopathic or additional homeopathic therapies—to the contrary, they enhance them. The placenta remedy quickly soothes nighttime bouts of coughing that accompany whooping cough.

Children who are treated with placenta remedies will have few symptoms with childhood diseases, yet after recovery they will have antibodies. Placenta globules eliminate symptoms such as fever, seizures and rashes, yet do not interfere with the child's immune process. The placenta pills provide a supplementary therapy, even if not given in time to prevent the disease entirely. The dosage is up to the judgment of the homeopathic practitioner.

Diseases of the Heart and Circulatory System

Heart attacks in women are not well understood and still not taken seriously enough. In addition, many women often do not have the severe pain that men do, and don't connect the fatigue, weakness, shortness of breath and dizziness with a heart attack—and neither do their physicians.(65)

Currently more women than men are dying from cardiovascular

disease. In the US and Canada it is the leading cause of death for women and men. In addition to elevated lipoproteins in the blood, heart attacks are exacerbated by high blood pressure, diabetes, obesity, job-related stress, lack of exercise and cigarette-smoking. According to Professor Eberhard Windler from the University of Eppendorf, "the pathogenic changes of the blood vessels start very early, roughly at the age of 13, and slowly progress unnoticed."(66)

After menopause a woman's risk of having a heart attack rises dramatically. The drop in estrogen can lead to increased blood pressure, weight gain and diminished stress tolerance, likely caused by inadequate adaptation to stress.(67)

Placenta products can be used as a source of protective hormones for cardiovascular diseases such as heart attacks and strokes, or after heart surgery.

Placenta remedies could even have a preventive function in national health, considering the large number of people suffering from strokes and their aftereffects.

A stroke may be treated with a remedy such as placenta cream, placenta extract or placenta powder. Even the precursors of a stroke may be influenced by placenta remedies; lack of concentration and motivation, depression and loss of appetite all respond well to placenta remedies according to a clinical double-blind study on 105 elderly patients at the hospital for senior citizens in Nürnberg.(68)

English scientists have discovered that estrogen has a direct relaxing effect on the coronary vessels and dilates the vessels of the periphery during attacks of angina pectoris.(69) Hutton, et. al. came to the conclusion that the extract of the placenta also prevents the clotting of blood platelets.(70)

These combined effects on the dilation of the vessels and viscosity of the blood may help avoid infarct and stroke. The placental hormones inhibit the hypothalamic feedback to stress, thus reducing the perception of stress and balancing geriatric mood swings.

The tissue of the placenta contains estrogens, which lower cholesterol, as well as prostaglandins and enzymes that influence the blood vessels, all of which positively affect cardiovascular diseases.(71) Placenta remedies are well-suited for preventing coronary and vascular diseases while being easily accessible and optimally composed for the human being. Substances proven to be part of the placenta extract are vitamins, hormones, lipids, cations, anions, amino acids, ferments and their components like creatinine, glucose and blood urea nitrogen. The placenta has effects similar to those of adrenocorticotrophic hormone (ACTH) and cortisol.(72)

For all these reasons, having individual homeopathic remedies made from one's own placenta as a medicine for prevention and family use is sensible. A laboratory that specializes in producing medicine from organic raw materials, in a country where it is legal, can be asked to potentiate the placental tissue. Doctors and health care practitioners frequently use standardized and sterilized commercial pharmacological products in their patients' therapies, including treatment for congestive heart failure, peripheral vascular disorders and high blood pressure. Placenta remedies can be added to the list of such therapies.

Menopause and Midlife Conditions

Osteoporosis

Osteoporosis is a common chronic disease, affecting 55% of people over the age of 50, 80% of whom are women.(73) This painful and crippling disease leads to brittle bones that break easily. Consumption of vitamin D and calcium, performing regular weight-bearing exercise and muscle training, which increase muscle mass and improve balance, and not smoking can slow bone loss. Estrogen, which also alleviates other symptoms older women have, as well as bisphosphonates and selector estrogen receptor modulators are drugs most frequently used in treatment.(74)

Hormone Replacement

Menopause (the time when the ovaries stop functioning after a woman's fertile lifespan) usually occurs between the ages of 40 and 58. A woman's average life expectancy currently is 79.7 years. Many women take hormone replacement therapy (HRT) during these years. Often a short period of treatment is all they need to deal with the uncomfortable side-effects experienced during menopause. In the past few years, however, studies have shown that the adverse effects of HRT outweigh the benefits. While HRT can help prevent bone fractures, it can also increase the risk for heart disease and cancer.

"The balance between the risks and the benefits of hormone treatment varies, depending on the length of treatment," says Francine Godstein, an internist of the gynecological clinic in Boston, who was in charge of a study asking 122,000 nurses every two years about their habits, diet and health.(75) In addition to the problems with side effects of hormones, she discovered that finding the correct individual dosage is difficult. Placenta remedies contain both estrogen and progesterone in their biological concentration produced by the human body itself. They might be suitable as a substitute for hormone therapies.

The placenta remedies with a high potency, in particular, may have positive effects on menopausal symptoms. These remedies may influence calcium metabolism in the bones if osteoporosis sets in after menopause. Calcium still must be made available to the body through nutrition, however.

Calcium is one of the most important components for building bones and teeth. As a component of the body's cells, the intracellular substance and the blood, calcium is essential for many vital processes; for example, blood clotting. It enhances the activity of the white blood cells and therefore raises the resistance to infections, soothes the central nervous system and counter-balances the stimulation of the muscles. Side-effects of osteoporosis, which can be caused by of a lack of calcium, can be treated with placenta substances. Taking the homeopathic placenta remedy for approximately three months should improve bone density.

Dementia

According to a large study in the Netherlands, the incidence of dementia in men and women has been found to be similar, although after age 90 the incidence decreases in men.(76) In some cases, Alzheimer's, one cause of dementia, is believed to have a genetic link.(77)

Considering that women make up the majority of the older population, we have to realize that the three most important areas of geriatric medicine in the future will be osteoporosis, cardiovascular disease and dementia.

Some women may experience psychiatric symptoms such as confusion, depression, paranoid psychosis and a failing short-term memory after menopause. Many are treated with psychotropic drugs or even hospitalized because hormone treatment was not sufficient. Placenta therapy can be an alternative for these patients, also avoiding the problem of dependency on certain drugs. Many women are particularly comfortable with the idea of using the placenta of one of their grandchildren.

In an acute situation a high dose of the female sex hormones is appropriate. An initial dosage of placenta powder or a vaginal suppository made of dried placenta may be useful in improving the acute symptoms. Long-term therapy combining high potencies of placenta should follow. The woman should take alternating high and low potencies of the placenta remedy in order to get her body to regulate the release of hormones properly again. Her vitality may be reestablished through this regimen.

Experience has shown that symptoms of aging such as wrinkles, loss of hair or the phenomenon of "dry eye" are the first to disappear; after about two months of treatment the cardiovascular and immune systems and memory improve. To maintain this health status the patient should continue taking the placenta remedy in longer intervals until she has been completely healed—approximately six months.

TCM recommends a cooling raw placenta remedy to balance hyperthyroid-caused symptoms. The body can adapt to the new hormonal situation of post menopause, with deficiencies counterbalanced.

Hair Loss and Scalp Problems

As previously mentioned, placenta remedies are used to treat some types of baldness and seborrhea.
(Note: See chapter II for discussion of adverse effects from use of placenta in cosmetics.)

In many patients, hair loss results from long-term inflammation of the scalp or from a nutritional deficiency. The main therapeutic goal for any type of hair loss is to substitute nutrients relevant to hair growth.

Assessment of the contents of the placenta extract will help in understanding the scale of possibilities for its use locally: the extract contains proteins, enzymes, vitamins, amino acids, nucleotides and mucopolysaccharides whose effectiveness have been proven by dermo-cosmetic tests. Particularly in the area around the hair follicles, the active substances of the placenta develop their normalizing effect on disorders of the blood flow to the scalp. This improves the nutrition and oxygenation of the cells of the hair follicles. This biostimulating effect seems to come mostly from the presence of glycosaminoglycan (mucopolysaccharide), which is abundant in the placenta extract.

Experience has shown that simply rubbing the placenta on the hairless spot will not suffice. Heat is necessary to improve the blood circulation and allow the amino acids and mucopolysaccharides to develop their effect. Thin hair will become fuller and shinier with the use of placenta extract. Structurally defective hair will become healthy and stronger from within. Three weeks of three to four applications per week are recommended for treating hair loss. This should be followed by at least one application per week. Placenta therapy reliably reduces the loss of hair and simultaneously makes the scalp healthier and tighter.

After the hair has been washed, an extract from the placenta (78) is put on the scalp. (See hair conditioner [spirunzenta] on page 60.) The scalp is then stimulated with a massage and an infrared lamp until the skin becomes slightly pinkish and feels warm. This heat, along with the increased blood circulation, allows the skin to absorb the placenta remedy. The hair growth will resume only a few days later.

Skin Conditions

Placenta remedies are particularly effective on skin problems. Various products available commercially contain proteins derived from the placenta. Most of them are from animal products, predominantly sheep and cows, however. Many customers who disapprove of these products appreciate homemade skin care products made with their own placenta substances.

One active substance in the placenta is the hormone

progesterone. It inhibits the breakdown of collagen in the skin. As we age, our natural collagen breaks down, leading to wrinkles. This process can be stopped with placenta ointments or by taking placenta remedies orally. The progesterone will stimulate the protein synthesis of the hormones, including relaxin. The hormone relaxin reestablishes the strength of the collagen in skin, bones and ligaments.

In addition to the progesterone, the placenta contains a lot of estrogen, which builds collagen. After approximately two months of treatment the skin will look fresh and smooth again. The rejuvenation and tightening of the skin is mostly a result of these two components of the natural multi-component-remedy placenta.

Dehydroepiandrosterone (DHEA), a natural steroid prohormone, and cortisols of the placenta help to heal infected skin. Parents in France have known of this effect since the 17th century.(79)

Side effects comparable to those from a cortisone treatment are not to be expected since the placenta only contains preliminary forms of this hormone. The cortex of the renal gland is therefore not affected by the cortisol in a placenta remedy.

Placenta ointment (see recipe on page 52) is a particularly effective vehicle for treating skin diseases. Within only a few minutes of application the placenta ointment will diminish the symptoms of inflammatory skin diseases as well as non-specific itching.

A newborn's diaper rash will respond just as quickly as an elderly person's itchy skin. The ointment can also be used for gestational pruritus (an insatiable itch during pregnancy, most commonly related to liver problems).

Patients with atopic dermatitis believe these ointments work faster if they add the extract or powder from their own placenta. This results from the effect of the nosode.(80)

IV. FROM PLACENTA TO HEALING REMEDY

Pharmacopoea Wirtenbergica, Stuttgart ed. 1741-1771, Translation:

Preparation of Human Placenta
Take!
One human afterbirth
Take away skins and cord
Wipe away the blood
Wash in sufficient volume of wine
Cut into pieces
Dry gently
Store at a tepid location

It is usually powdered for difficult births.
The dosage is one Skrupel to a half Drachme (around 1.2-1.8 gram)

Methods of Preservation

A mature placenta with the full complement of enzymes, fats, hormones and blood cells is nutritious tissue, not only for humans but for other forms of life such as germs, molds and insects. To keep it longer than five days you must preserve it by cooking, drying or sterilization.

Like the Germans of the 17th century, the Chinese boil the placenta in water and use both the placenta and the water for making the various placenta remedies. The most well-known recipe is postpartum soup, made from a small piece of the placenta and chicken or beef soup.(81) The stock is mostly used for injections and tinctures. In TCM, cooking is an integral part of the formation and action of the medicine. Steaming at a low temperature is meant to enrich the placenta with energy. After cooking it is powdered or put in capsules (82) for a convenient application (see recipe for placenta capsules on page 55).

Another method is the mummification of the placenta as in the Egyptian tradition. The placenta is dried in the sun or the oven until it is hard and crumbly. If the placenta was infected with yeast the drying process will sterilize it. Chunks of the placenta are then ground, processed in a mortar and further processed into a powder.

Occasionally, when the child has meconium-stained amniotic fluid, the placenta may be infected. The amniotic fluid has a tendency to take in pathogenic germs, which can render the placenta useless for healing. An infected placenta can be treated by sterilization.

To sterilize the placenta before mummification put a shallow glass pan of vinegar water under the placenta in the oven. At a temperature of 160°F (70° C) the vapor from the vinegar will kill the germs within an hour. No reaction to the vinegar vapor is expected because the drying process draws the water out of the placenta. The vinegar-vapor-process is a gentle sterilization method for biological substances against spores, bacteria and viruses.(83)

Both raw and fresh tissue can be used for healing purposes as well. The placenta can be kept fresh in the refrigerator for five days; after that it needs to be frozen. Although freezing the placenta destroys the B vitamins, the hormones and many other components stay intact.

Fresh Placenta

Prior to preservation, the placenta can be used as a whole for the treatment of a skin disorder. After preservation the tissue should be used only for external treatments.

The fresh placenta can be used as a healing compress for a family member with atopic dermatitis. Place the maternal side of the placenta on the afflicted skin. The patient will immediately feel warmth, which moves from that part of the skin through the entire body. Sometimes the sense of heat may be as intense as a burn. The change of temperature in the skin can also be felt on the other side of the placenta with the amniotic membranes—the placenta itself will become hot. After a little while the placenta will seem cold and its beneficial effect is over. Remove the placenta from the skin and carefully dry the area. The sore from the dermatitis will have dried up and the redness will be gone.

Even moles, birthmarks and skin cancer are said to have been treated in this manner in the 17th century. In his *Dictionnaire des Drogues*, Nicolas Lemery reports in 1697: For the moles to disappear, the placenta has to be placed on the face as long as it is still warm, immediately after it comes from the uterus.(84) In the meantime more agreeable methods such as pulverized placenta and placenta-containing creams have been developed to heal skin defects.

Even today in some countries women customarily eat parts of the raw placenta (placentophagia) within hours after giving birth. The tissue of the placenta is said to be so nutritious that they have little appetite for other food. This custom is said to aid in the involution of the uterus to normal size and to establish the milk supply more quickly. Two other effects of placentophagia are "accelerated onset of maternal behavior" and enhancement of pain relief.(85)

The custom of eating the placenta is currently going through a revival among some women in the US and other countries. As a result, these women have tested various ways of preparing the raw placenta.

Some women eat a piece of the raw placenta postpartum, after washing it in salty water and refrigerating it. The frozen piece is cut into very thin slices and the woman ingests one of them each day.

Other women swallow two capsules of placenta tissue three times a day.(86) Others eat the placenta pieces, which have been kept fresh in the refrigerator, on their breakfast rolls with onions and salt. Scalded slices of the placenta are also eaten for dinner along with boiled vegetables. Some women have compared the taste to that of steak tartare (a meat dish made from finely chopped or ground raw beef). Even vegetarians claim that they don't dislike the taste of their placentas.

> ### How to Process a Homeopathic Mother Tincture
>
> Remove a small finger-nail sized bit of placenta tissue from the middle of the placenta with a scalpel or scissors. Put this small piece of placenta into a bowl and crush it until mushy. Add pure fresh or filtered water and stir with figure eight movements or in one direction until the water becomes funnel-shaped; then stir in the opposite direction. Strain the essence through a cheesecloth. Take 10 ml of this mixture and add 90 ml fresh water, swing it in a covered glass jar in figure eight. (Note: 10 ml is equivalent to approximately seven tablespoons.) After 50 swings, fix the medium by clapping on the bottom of the glass, and strain again.
>
> Repeat by taking 10 ml of the strained essence and adding 90 ml of water; then perform the same procedure with swinging and fixing the solution. Do this three or four times and fix with medical alcohol. (In Germany the D3 (third dilution) is the first potency you are allowed to give out, if the origin was not herbal.) This mother-tincture is ready for a homeopathy laboratory to produce higher potencies, because the purity is guaranteed to not transmit any diseases.

Frozen Placenta

To heal sore nipples, a slice of raw, frozen placenta may be placed on the fissure. This dressing will accelerate the healing process to the point that nursing is possible again in time for the baby's next feeding. Any residues of the placenta tissue on the nipples will not harm the baby, since it does not contain any foreign protein. To the contrary, the baby is particularly fond of the oxytocin in the tissue of the placenta. Oxytocin is contained in the mother's milk, as well, and makes the hard work of sucking more enjoyable. A placenta dressing is the ideal remedy for fissures and sore nipples.

When using the placenta for this purpose, wash it in salt water to rinse off any blood and then freeze it. Cut a slice as thin as the blade of a knife and place on the wound as a dressing.

The blood-clotting particles such as fibrinogen and thrombocytic fractions will cause scrapes, fissures and cuts, as well as sutured and closed wounds, to develop a new layer of skin and lose the swelling more quickly. The net of fibrinogen in the tissue of the placenta keeps germs from spreading and accelerates the proliferation of cells within the wound. With a placenta dressing a wound can completely heal within only a few hours.

Drying the Placenta

The most practical method of processing the placenta is to dry it. This method has been and still is being used all over the world. Depending on the culture, the placenta is dried in the oven or in the sun. When the placenta is finally mummified after many hours, it will still need to be protected from bacteria and insects.

Traditionally the dried placenta is wrapped in a piece of cloth and hung in a cool, dry place to be cured like bacon. In a modern household, a preferable method is to grind it into a powder and keep it in a well-sealed jar in the refrigerator. The powder can then be used to produce various remedies.

The placenta must be completely mummified before being pulverized. The average placenta is 25 mm thick, has a diameter of 22 cm and weighs about 500 g. Depending on the size and thickness of the organ, an average of three days and three nights is required for it to dry enough to be broken into chunks.

The exposure to heat during the drying process should be as gentle on the healing substances as possible. Afterwards, the placenta will only be half its original size and will have turned hard and black. It needs to be brittle enough to be crushed into pieces with a heavy object.

First, grate the dry chunks of placenta, then grind with a coffee mill or with a mortar and pestle. Keep removing the powder and grinding the bigger pieces. If the powder is still not fine enough, add a carrier substance such as sugar, silica or mineral earth. The crystals of the carrier substance will make the powder even finer.

The completed placenta powder keeps best in a cool, dry place. The container should be marked with the date the powder was made, the dilution and the origin of the raw material. Experience shows that the powder can be stored for up to three years. If bacteria, spores or parasites are not destroyed, the powder will develop a bad smell. If this happens, do not use the powder anymore.

Further Processing of Placenta Powder

The placenta powder will dissolve immediately if you add an emulsifier such as ghee, lecithin or coconut emulsifier. This emulsion can be added to food, such as a milk product or bread spread containing fat. The dry powder and the emulsion have the same effects, but people's preferences vary.

The placenta emulsion (see recipe on p. 51) is also suitable for use as a bath additive. It can be used in the bath water to help relieve nervous exhaustion, problems with blood circulation, back pain or nerve pain. The temperature of the bath water depends on personal tolerance and should be between 98.5°–102° F (37°C and 39°C). Higher temperatures intensify the effect. A health care professional should prescribe the application. If fever, severe heart disease, a circulatory system disorder or high blood pressure is present, the health practitioner should determine whether a placenta bath is indicated and the correct dosage.

Doctors and naturopaths have also found placenta baths helpful for headaches, heart problems in elderly people and brachial plexus neuritis (shoulder-arm-syndrome).

The placenta emulsion also provides a good base for making placenta ointments. For the treatment of skin disorders, choose a suitable carrier oil. Good choices include avocado oil, meadowfoam seed oil or a medium chain triglyceride (MCT) because these oils are well absorbed even by sensitive skin. Adding placenta emulsion to ointments that contain cortisol can significantly increase their effect. Eucerin Aquaphor ointment seems to be the least irritating for particularly sensitive people. The appropriate carrier oil for the ointment should be chosen individually for each patient.

Finely ground placenta powder can be used for ointments for various therapies. Research on intracellular tissue space shows that a number of substances can pass through the epidermis (the tough layer of skin on the body's surface) by diffusion. In addition, epithelializing layers of cells serve as a storage space. This means creams and ointments can pass an even dosage on to the deeper layers of the skin for hours and days.

The lower layers of the skin are crisscrossed by blood and lymph vessels. These vessels absorb the substances and transport them farther, making possible a systemic effect (87) without the risk of overdose or undesirable hormonal effects.

Placenta powder added to an ointment is a good treatment for diaper rash, as well. The redness will disappear immediately and inflamed areas will heal within only a few hours. The ointment works particularly quickly right after a warm bath since the softened skin allows the substances to be more readily absorbed.

Pregnant women suffering from gestational pruritus often

prefer the dermatitis ointment or ghee (see recipe on page 51). If no immediate improvement occurs, the effect can be enhanced by heating the skin with infrared light.

Combining the use of placenta ointments with other therapeutic measures that raise the temperature of the skin is highly recommended. This reduces the viscosity of the skin's fat and allows lipophilic substances to dissolve more readily. The enlarged capillaries and vessels of the skin speed up the transport of the substances. In other words, the ointments work particularly well after a warm bath, underneath a pillow of dried wild flowers or with infrared light.(88)

Application of Placenta Globules

This list is of applications that have been collected and used by young families with common medical problems. Some midwives, naturopaths and pediatricians have integrated the placenta remedies into their treatment. Ask about them when consulting a practitioner.

D6	Improving breast milk, when baby grows or is dissatisfied	1x 2-3 globules
D8/C7	Baby w/flu, cough, stuffy nose	2-3 globules, not after 2 pm
D12	Pains prior to/during menses	3x daily 2 globules, start 3 days before
D20	Regulating menstrual cycle, "Male Potency" for vertebra/knee diseases	1x daily from ovulation day, male take 5-15 glob. daily
D30	Baby with indigestion/not nursing	1x 2globule
D30	Prevents distress at baptism, family events, doctor visit, etc.	1x 2globules for baby/mother
D30	Severe, persistent flu, cough, following D8 application, comb with other homeopathy	1x daily 2 globules
D30	Childhood diseases, menopausal, geriatric, skin disorders, dry eye	2-3x daily 7globules

V. RECIPES FOR THE MEDICINE CABINET

Placenta Ghee (Mother Butter)

3½ oz butter (100 g)
1 teaspoon placenta powder
jar for 3½ oz of ointment (100 g)
essential oil of choice (optional)

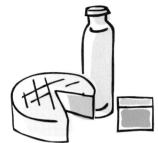

Melt the butter and skim off the foam while allowing it to simmer on the stove. Then add placenta powder and stir.

Let the mixture set for approximately five hours in the oven or on the stove at 120°–140° F (50°–60° C). Stir until the powder has dissolved, using a blender if necessary. Pour the mixture into a jar. Let it cool at room temperature, not in the refrigerator. Store in the refrigerator for up to four weeks.

Variation: Depending on personal preferences and sensitivity of the skin, a drop of essential oil can be added. The somewhat disagreeable odor of placenta will improve with an essential oil of lemongrass, ylang-ylang and others.

Placenta Emulsion

1/3 oz emulsifier (10 g)
1 oz distilled water (30 ml)
1/2 tsp of placenta powder (2 g)

Dissolve the emulsifier in distilled water at 120° F (50° C). Add placenta powder as soon as the solution has turned into a paste. Simmer at the same temperature while stirring swiftly, until the powder has dissolved completely. Remove from heat and let soak. Cool at room temperature while beating it well with a whisk.

Placenta Ointment

¾ tsp placenta powder (3 g)
1 tsp carrier oil (almond, meadowfoam seed, avocado)
1½ oz Eucerin Aquaphor ointment (45 g)

Heat oil together with the placenta powder to 120° (50° C). Use a blender to dissolve the powder until the grains are as fine as possible. Cool to 98.5° F (37° C) and mix in the Aquaphor ointment. Let it set until completely cooled. Can be stored for three weeks.

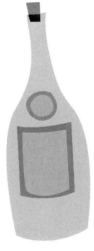

Placenta Tincture (Mother Essence)

2 cups 40% alcohol (1/2 liter)
2 cups isotone saline solution (0.9%) (1/2 liter)
1 piece placenta, thumbnail size
1 dark glass bottle and matching cork
1 firm piece of cloth
sun or warmth

Cut a piece the size of a thumbnail from the placenta. Wash it in the salt water and put the piece in a dark sterilized bottle. Pour in the alcohol and seal bottle with a thick piece of cloth. Put the bottle in the sun or keep it in a warm room. Pour the tincture into a sterile bottle after 24 hours (without the placenta piece). Seal with a clean cork.

Placenta Bath

2 oz placenta emulsion (50 g)
1 cup warm water

Mix the placenta emulsion with the warm water. Mix in a blender until it is foamy, then add to bath water.

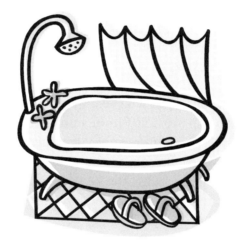

Lactation Drink

1 generous pinch placenta powder
1 glass of at least lukewarm beer or champagne

Sprinkle placenta powder into the beer or champagne and allow to foam. To keep the foam from spilling, the glass should be twice as tall as the liquid content. Drink in little sips and the production of milk will be stimulated within 20 minutes. (This works best with dark beer and works great even without the powder!)

Lactation Soup

2 cups tomato puree (1/2 liter)
1 generous pinch of paprika powder
1–2 onions, cut into quarters
1 teaspoon Kombu algae powder
1 teaspoon placenta powder
3 tablespoons olive oil
2–3 squid
2–3 different kinds of fish fillets
sea salt, water, white wine

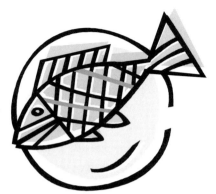

Combine squid, onions, spices, algae and placenta powders, and tomato puree and bring to a boil. Simmer until the squid is tender. Add water and wine. Once it has stopped boiling, carefully place the fish filet in the soup. Be sure not to stir the soup again! This soup supplies the mother with the seafood protein needed to make her milk. The placenta stimulates the milk-producing glands.

Raw Placenta Pills

placenta
freezer
saw knife

Clean the placenta on a cookie sheet, cutting off membranes and cord, and put it into the freezer.

After several hours, cut with a sharp knife into thin slices and put them in single layers into a container. Every day mother should swallow one frozen placenta pill one hour before eating.

Placenta Capsules

whole placenta
2 cups fresh water (1/2 liter)
2 fresh ginger slices
½ lemon
1 pinch hot pepper
steamer
food dehydrator
"00"capsules
coffee grinder

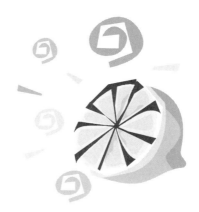

To cook the placenta, wash excess blood off and wrap bloody side inside the membranes. Place in a steamer over water. Combine ginger, lemon and hot pepper; add placenta. Steam for 15 minutes over low heat. Turn placenta and steam 15 more minutes until no juice comes out when pricked with a fork. After steaming, slice placenta into thin strips. Place strips on a cookie sheet in the oven on lowest possible setting for several hours until completely dry and brittle. (Using a food dehydrator is even better, if placed outside on a balcony or terrace (smell!), but will take longer.) Powder the strips in a coffee grinder and put into capsules. These can be kept indefinitely, but are best kept in an airtight container in the freezer long-term.(89)

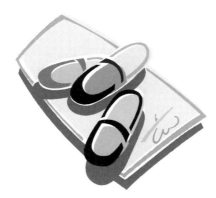

German Postpartum Soup

1 lb beef (500 g)
1 leek, cut in slices
additional soup vegetables
1 teaspoon placenta, either raw or pulverized
½ gallon water (2 liters)
1 cup cream (1/4 liter)
3-4 eggs
1/2 cup of wine (1/8 liter)
salt, saffron, nutmeg

Cook the meat with the placenta and the vegetables (except the leek) in the water until meat is tender. Remove from heat. Add the leek and cream. Next add wine and the spices according to taste. Beat the eggs separately and then gently stir them into the soup. Garnish the soup with chopped fresh herbs to taste.

Recipe from the 18th century

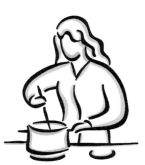

Placenta Soup

4 cups water (1 liter)
1 thumbnail size piece of placenta
1 tablespoon Miso optional)
chicken parts, vegetables, spices, bunch of herbs

Combine the chicken parts with the vegetables and spices and boil them in the water. Just before the chicken and vegetables are done, add the placenta piece. Take soup off the heat after several minutes and let cool to 122° F (50° C). Stir in the herbs. Vegetarians can leave out the chicken and add cold pressed vegetable oil and Miso instead.

Placenta Cream

2 oz Rescue or Five-Flower-Ointment (50 g)
3 drops placenta tincture (mother essence)
Warm the ointment in a water bath and stir in the placenta mother tincture. Let set for several days before using.

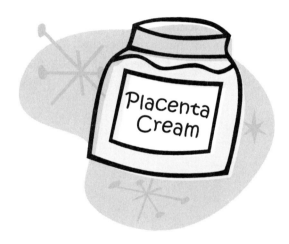

Placenta Foot Ointment

1/3 oz placenta emulsion (10 g)
3 tablespoons silica gel

After making the placenta emulsion let it cool to 98.5° F. (37° C). Combine with the silica gel and let it hydrate. Apply ointment in between toes and wash off after two hours. Dry toes completely with a blow dryer. You may want to apply a layer of placenta cream afterwards.

Placenta Dressing

raw placenta tissue
isotonic saline solution
gauze

Cut a piece from the fresh placenta, following the natural grooves. Wash in saline solution and conserve in the freezer. Cut a slice from the frozen placenta tissue. (Cut as thin as possible.) Place this cooling slice on the closed wound. Cover with gauze or a soft, absorbent material. Leave the dressing on the wound for approximately half an hour. Destroy the placenta tissue after use.

Compress

1 stick butter (125 g)
1 teaspoon finely ground placenta powder
cotton cloth
absorbent cotton
flannel
hot water bottle

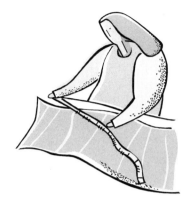

Heat the butter and skim off foam. Add placenta powder and stir at 120° F (50° C) until the powder dissolves. (Use a blender if necessary.) Cut two layers from the cotton cloth in the desired size. Cover with a thick layer of absorbent cotton and then place a somewhat larger piece of flannel on top.

Let the first cotton layer soak up the placenta butter until fabric is saturated. Allow to cool to 100° F (36–38° C), then place it on the painful area. Cover with the prepared absorbent cotton–flannel compress and put the hot water bottle on top to keep the ingredients liquid. Keep the compress in place for roughly half an hour and destroy afterwards.

Nursing Oil (Placentolact)

2/3 oz placenta emulsion (20 g)
1/3 cup apricot seed oil (85 ml)
1 drop geranium essential oil *(Pelargonium graveolens)*

Prepare placenta emulsion. Once it has cooled, add the apricot seed oil and the geranium essential oil, giving it an inviting fragrance. Apply to the breast and the lymphatic ducts after each feeding, avoiding the nipples. Use only once a day if milk supply is good.

Baby Care Paste

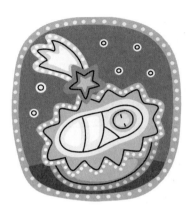

½ oz emulsifier (15 g)
1 oz almond oil (30 g)
1/3 oz placenta powder (10 g)
1/3 oz shea butter (10 g)
1 oz water (30 ml)

Stirring constantly, heat the emulsifier, almond oil and shea butter to a maximum of 130° F (55° C). Add the placenta powder and stir until granules are dissolved. Let the mixture cool. Heat water to 160° F (70° C) in another pan. Reheat the mixture of oil and butter to 160° F (70° C), as well. Gradually add the hot water to the mixture while stirring briskly. Allow to cool at room temperature. Drain or mix in any water separating from the mixture.

Hair Conditioner (Spiruzenta)

1 oz placenta emulsion (30 g)
1-2/3 oz Spirulina powder (50 g)
2/3 oz distilled water (20 ml)

Dilute fresh placenta emulsion with the distilled water and stir in Spirulina powder. Allow to hydrate. Apply the paste to hairless areas and cover with a plastic cap/hood. Expose area to infrared lamp for at least 30 minutes. Wash hair after each application. Use twice a week.

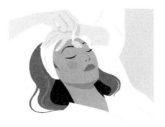

Facial Mask (Plastevia-Saluber)

1 part placenta powder
1 part stevia powder
2 parts mineral earth
2 parts water

Combine placenta powder and stevia powder. Prepare mineral earth, add the powder and apply the paste to any itching, inflamed, sore or cracked areas of the skin. Allow mask to dry for up to a maximum of 15 minutes and remove with a moist cloth. Rinse with plenty of lukewarm water. If desire, apply placenta ointment afterwards.

Placenta Drink

piece of fresh placenta
apple juice, ½ banana, etc...

Verena Schmid

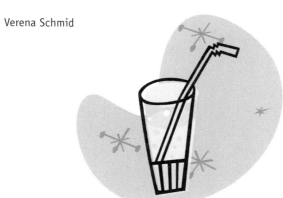

VI. WOMEN TELL THEIR STORIES

Does a Placenta Smell Appetizing?

When I was pregnant I first heard of the option of eating the placenta and thought it was totally disgusting. But a growing number of newspaper reports, stories from other women and my midwives' advice made me curious.

I was concerned I might not be able to breastfeed well, since I was already bothered by swollen legs when I was in the 22nd week of pregnancy. So I decided to consume my raw placenta. Because I was disgusted with the thought, a friend recommended I cut five thin slices off the placenta and put them in the freezer. I did so. This way I even had enough placenta left over to plant an apple tree for our baby.

When my baby was born, the midwife showed the placenta to me and we talked about which part might be tasty. Suddenly everything had changed—what an odd consideration! The entire placenta smelled tasty and I couldn't imagine how in the world the placenta could have been something disgusting to me up until then. I proudly asked my friend who had assisted at the birth if she smelled it as well. She only said: "Well, yes, it does have a unique smell to it!"

I immediately tested a small piece after it was rinsed off with salt water and presented to me by my husband in a salami sandwich. He could not picture me wanting it without the camouflaging sandwich. But I picked the slice of placenta out of the sandwich, put it straight into my mouth and was surprised to find out it tasted like Tartare.

Where can you still eat Tartare anymore these days—it was great! This, to my surprise, satisfied my appetite and I didn't need anything to eat for the next 24 hours. We put five more slices in the freezer. Who knows, I might need the placenta again some time!

While I was eating the placenta piece my friend told me how embarrassed she had felt, when the placenta was shown to her after the birth of her child and it had seemed so appetizing. And it bothered her even more, that the placenta had simply been discarded in the garbage. Had she known back then that it was not at all unnatural "to like your placenta so much you could munch on it," she would not have let that happen.

We realized that it is apparently only the mother (and maybe the baby?) to whom the smell of the placenta is appealing. Why had I been so disgusted with it before? I conclude that I am not supposed to eat anybody else's placenta, but my very own had definitely invited me to do so! In any case it presented me with a flourishing dairy and a very content baby.

Heidi G. from Mühlhausen, Germany

Home Treatment for the Colicky Baby

Since I was repeatedly depressed during pregnancy I didn't expect things to be easy after the birth. I decided to have homeopathic pills made from the placenta. My health care practitioner had the pills made and he was there for me for consultation at any given time.

I was glad I hardly needed the pills at all. I had a quiet and quick homebirth in water and had no postpartum depression whatsoever. Instead, the baby was very restless and cried for two hours straight every evening. It was gaining weight well and showed no symptoms of illness, so nobody knew how to help. Finally it got to the point where the whole family was upset and my husband made a decision: We had heard the pills could help the baby as well. So the stressed father ordered a treatment with the children's potency C7, three pills every hour from 5:00 pm to 8:00 pm.

Already the very first night was definitely quieter. Our baby cried with less intensity, nursed for a longer period and went back to sleep within only an hour. We assumed the dosage had been correct and kept giving the placenta pills to the baby every night. And, abracadabra— within two weeks the spell was gone—no more wailing, no more crying.

The midwife, asking us for the cause of the wonderful transformation of our baby, encouraged our autonomous treatment. We had probably influenced the stress hormones with the placenta nosode. She also recommended that we take the baby to baby swimming classes, since the water can help the child find its own equilibrium. And indeed, our baby was thrilled about the water and from six weeks on became the most faithful pool-visitor of our region. The siblings came along and the entire family enjoyed our waterbaby. The crying spells that had occurred in the beginning were long forgotten.

With our next baby we will pay attention to the stresses it might be exposed to beginning with pregnancy. But since my environment never spoiled me during my pregnancies, I will have placenta pills made again, just in case. They were a great help for all of us.

Irene M. from Enzweihingen, Germany

VII. REFERENCES

1. Scholl, Michael. Baldwin Midwife Wages Legal Battle to Upend Suspension of Privileges. *New York Law Journal*, 17 Oct 2006.
2. Lauer, Nancy Cook. Hawaiian Law Now Permits Parents to Keep Placentas. *Womensense News*, 28 Jul 2006.
3. Campe, Joachim Heinrich. 1809. Wörterbuch der deutschen Sprache, Braunschweig.
4. Eggert, Barbara. 1986. Untersuchungen zur Ethnographie der Geburt am Beispiel Indonesien. *Magisterarbeit München*.
5. Gélis, Jacques. 1992. Das Geheimnis der Geburt. Herder, Freiburg.
6. Muehlstegen, Inka. 1993. The Midwifery Consciousness of Placenta, Deutsche Hebammenzeitung.
7. Dowling, Terence. 1992. Prenatal Placenta Symbiosis and Its Meaning for Parenting. Lecture on ISSPM-Congress. Oct 1992
8. Strauss, M. Von der Zeichensprache des kleinen Kindes, Stuttgart 1977
9. See note 4 above.
10. See note 8 above.
11. Hesse, Hermann. 1986. *Das Glassperlenspiel*, Vester F: Ein Baum ist mehr als ein Baum, Koesel Muenchen.
12. Dunham, Carroll. 1992. *Mamatoto—A Celebration of Birth*, London: Virago Press.
13. See note 5 above.
14. See note 9 above.
15. Vescoli, Michael. 1995. *Der Keltische Baumkalender (The Celtic Tree Calendar)*, Muenchen.
16. *Glassperienspiel*..
17. Raetsch, Chr. 1998. *Hexenmedizin (Medicine of the Hags)*. AT-Verlag Aarau/CH.
18. *Mamatoto*.
19. See note 5 above.
20. See note 4 above.
21. See note 5 above.
22. Jueptner, H. 1986. Geburtshilflich-gynaekologische Beobachtungen bei den Trobriandern *Obstet Gynecol* (Observations of Trobriander Sonderband Curare.)
23. Braun, G.K. 1959. Untersuchungen ueber das Brauchtum um Schwangerschaft und Geburt (Investigations of pregnancy and birth customs), Dissertation Uni Koeln.
24. See note 2 above.
25. Ibid.
26. Ibid.
27. Ibid.
28. *Mamatoto*.
29. Rademacher, R. and D. Rademacher. Waidelich. 1996. Nachweise fuer den rituellen Umgang mit Nachgeburten (Archeological prove of rites with placenta), Fundberichte Baden-Wuerttemberg 21.
30. Rademacher, R. 1991. ZUR Deutung von Funden neuzeitlicher Henkeltoepfe, Stadtarchiv Sindelfingen, Germany.
31. Historische Gesellschaft Boennigheim. 1997. Wo weder Sonne noch Mond hinscheint (Where nor sun nor moon shines), Stuttgart, Germany.
32. Drossel, D. 1997. Plazentatoepfe, Ludwigsburger Kreiszeitung.
33. Bohnenberger, K. 1904. Volkstuemliche Ueberlieferungen in Baden-Wuerttemberg, Stuttgart, Germany.
34. Loux, Francoise. 1959. Das Kind und sein Koerper in der Volksmedizin in Untersuchungen ueber das Brauchtum von Schwangerschaft und Geburt (s.12), Koeln, Germany.
35. Hoehn, H. *Sitte und Brauch bei Geburt, Taufe und in der Kindheit* (Customs and traditions at birth, baptism and early childhood) in Forschungen und Berichte zur Volkskunde in Baden-Wuerttemberg, vol.5.
36. Sheikh-Dilthey, H. Schwangerschaft und Geburt bei den indoarabischen Gruppen der Swahili-Kueste (Pregnancy and birth in Indoarab groups at Swahili Coast) in Schievenhoevel und Sich: Die Geburt aus ethnomedizinischer Sicht, Vieweg-Verlag Wiesbaden
37. *Mamatoto*.

38. Kludas, M. 1957. Die Plazenta-Therapie in der Weltliteratur in Therapiewoche.
39. Philipp, E. 1957. Die Hormone der Plazenta, Therapiewoche 79.
40. See note 5 above.
41. Ibid.
42. Ibid.
43. Ibid.
44. Becker, F. 1989. *Das passive Kreislauftraining-Das Frauenbad (The passive CVS Training- Womens´ Bath)*. Hamburg, Germany : Waerland Monatshefte.
45. Plazenta Human, Einfuehrung, Wiedemann Pharma GmbH, Muensing-Ambach 1989
46. Diamond, John. *Remothering—Das Wiedererleben der Mutterliebe*, Verlag f. Angewandte Kinesiologie, Freiburg 1991.
47. Ibid.
48. Odent, Michel. 1992. *The Nature of Birth and Breastfeeding*, London.
49. Ibid.
50. Odent, Michel. 2000. *Scientification of Love*. London.
51. www.powertoheal.com/Placenta%20Restorative%20Pills.htm. Accessed 16 Aug 2005.
52. www.minohonosaru.com/bitax/About_VITA_X.html. Accessed 20 Aug 2005.
53. Placental Histotherapy Center: History. www.histoterapia-placentaria.cu/informai.htm. Accessed 24 Oct 2006.
54. University of Texas, MD Anderson Cancer Center. Biologic/Organic/Pharmacologic Therapies: Govallo Placental extracts. www.mdanderson.org/departments/cimer/display.cfm?id=86407558-13ee-11d5-811000508b603a14&method=displayfull&pn=6eb86a59-ebd9-11d4-810100508b603a14. Accessed 18 Jul 2006.
55. Ibid.
56. Foulke, Judith E. Publication No. (FDA) 95-5013: *Cosmetic Ingredients: Understanding the Puffery*.U.S. Food and Drug Administration FDA Consumer magazine. May 1992.
57. Tiwary, C. 1998. Use of Estrogen- or Placenta-Containing Hair Products. *Clin Pediatr* 37: 733–40.
58. Maxwell, Nancy Irwin. 2000. Social Differences in Women's Use of Personal Care Products: Magazine Advertisements 1950-1994. http://library.silentspring.org/publications/pdfs/magazinestudy.pdf. Accessed 25 Oct 2006.
59. www.who.int/ethics/en/ETH_TissueBanking.pdf. Accessed 25 Oct 2006.
60. Personal correspondence from Alison Bastien, Jul 2006.
61. Kantkar, S.K. and C.P.Tewari. 1982. Human Placental Membrane as a Biological Dressing in Burns. *Indian Journal of Surgery*.
62. Schramm, Scluegg. 1900. Die Hausaerztin, Ehlers-Verlag St. Gallen/CH.
63. Lang, Raven. *Midwifery Today E-news*. July 2004, *Mothering* Sep 1983.
64. Lucziak, Hania. 2000. Das Zweite Gehirn (The Second Brain), *GEO-Magazine*.
65. McSweeney, J.C., et al. 2003. Women's Early Warning Symptoms of Acute Myocardial Infarction. *Circulation: Journal of the American Heart Association* http://usgovinfo.about.com/gi/dynamic/offsite.htm?zi=1/XJ&sdn=usgovinfo&zu=http%3A%2F%2Fcirc.ahajournals.org%2Fcgi%2Freprint%2F01.CIR.0000097116.29625.7Cv1. Accessed 30 Oct 2006.
66. Hamburger, Adenblatt. 147 vom 26 Jun 1996.
67. Lindholm, S.T., et al. 1992. Behavioural stress responses premenopausal, postmenopausal women and the effects of estrogen. *Am J Obstet Gynecol* 167(6): 1831–36.
68. Praxis Fibel Biomolekulare vit-Organ Therapie. 1994. Ostfildern, Germany.
69. Rosano, G.M., et al. 1993. Beneficial effect of oestrogen on exercise-induced myocardial ischaemia in women with coronary artery disease. *Lancet* 342(8864): 133–36.
70. Hutton, R.A., et al. 1980 Inhibition of platelet aggregation by placental extracts. *Thromb Res* 17(3–4): 465–71.
71. Karim, S. 1975. Physiological roles and pharmacological action of prostaglandins. In *Prostaglandins and Reproduction*. Lancaster: MTP
72. McLean, M., et al. 1995. A Placental Clock Controlling the Length of Human Pregnancy. *Nat Med* 1(5): 460–63.
73. National Osteoporosis Foundation. 2006. www.nof.org/osteoporosis/diseasefacts.htm. Accessed 26 Oct 2006.
74. Ibid.

75. Brown, David. Hormone Treatment: Only for a While? Washington Post Service, *Herald Tribune* 20 Jun 1997.
76. Neurobiol Aging 22(4): 575–80.
77. National Institute on Aging. Alzheimer's Disease Fact Sheet. www.nia.nih.gov/Alzheimers/Publications/adfact.htm. Accessed 26 Oct 2006.
78. Wevering, Trimbach. 1995. Einsatz der menschlichen Plazenta in der Trikologie (Application of placenta in human tricology, hair care) Wesel.
79. See note 34 above.
80. Cornelius, P. 1990. *Nosodentherapie*. Muenchen.
81. Bensky, D. and A Gamble. 1993. *Chinese Herbal Medicine-Materia* Medica. Seattle.
82. See note 63 above.
83. Theurer Karl. 1987. Innovative Biotherapie, Stuttgart, Germany.
84. See note 5 above.
85. Kristal, M.B. 1991. Enhancement of opioid-mediated analgesia: A solution to the enigma of placentophagia. *Neurosci Biobehav Rev* 15(3): 425–35.
86. See note 63 above.
87. Landsberger, A. 1994. Biologische Therapie ueber die Haut, Gotha, Germany.
88. Karl, J. 1994. Die Kombination von Plazentsalben mit physikalischen Therapien (Combination of placenta ointments with physiotherapies—Therapies through the skin) *Biologische Therapie ueber die Haut*, Gotha/Germany.
89. See note 63 above.

VIII. APPENDIX

Order form for laboratory work: (a)

_____

(name of laboratory)

Raw material for the preparation of nosodes:
Name of patient:_____
Date of birth:_____

The container holds a mixture suitable to store the raw material for further production of nosodes. Please make sure the container is marked correctly with name and date of birth.

    Put placenta tissue/sample—amount depending on availability but at a maximum pea size—without further manipulation inside tube.

The following potencies are desired (please mark):
- dilution
- globules
- (auto) nosode sequence (D6, D8, D12, D20, and D30 are suggested)
- mother tincture

Delivery address:

Billing address:

    (a) Choose a laboratory supervised by a pathologist and ask the lab for a container for your sample.

NOTES: